Vegan Diet

The Plan to Achieve the Keto-Vegetarian Lifestyle, to Burn Fat and Stimulate Your Energy

(Everyday Vegan Recipes and Clean Eating Meals)

Julio Barr

Published by Robert Satterfield Publishing House

© **Julio Barr**

All Rights Reserved

Vegan Diet Cookbook: The Plan to Achieve the Keto-Vegetarian Lifestyle, to Burn Fat and Stimulate Your Energy (Everyday Vegan Recipes and Clean Eating Meals)

ISBN 978-1-989787-26-7

All rights reserved. No part of this guide may be reproduced in any form without permission in writing from the publisher except in the case of brief quotations embodied in critical articles or reviews.

Legal & Disclaimer

The information contained in this book is not designed to replace or take the place of any form of medicine or professional medical advice. The information in this book has been provided for educational and entertainment purposes only.

The information contained in this book has been compiled from sources deemed reliable, and it is accurate to the best of the Author's knowledge; however, the Author cannot guarantee its accuracy and validity and cannot be held liable for any errors or omissions. Changes are periodically made to this book. You must consult your doctor or get professional medical advice before using any of the suggested remedies, techniques, or information in this book.

TABLE OF CONTENT

Part 1 1

Introduction 2

Chapter 1: Getting Started 5

WHAT IS VEGANISM? 5
WHAT IS THE DIFFERENCE BETWEEN VEGETARIANS AND VEGANS? 5
WHAT ARE THE DIFFERENT TYPES OF VEGANISM? 6
HEALTH VEGANISM: 6
ENVIRONMENTAL VEGANISM: 6
ETHICAL VEGANISM: 7
OTHERS: 8

Chapter 2: Important Questions 9

WHAT DOES THE VEGAN DIET INCLUDE? 9
WHAT DOES THE VEGAN DIET EXCLUDE? 9
HOW DO YOU SUBSTITUTE FOR DAIRY PRODUCTS? 10
ARE THERE ANY SUBSTITUTES FOR EGGS SUITABLE FOR MY VEGAN DIET? 12

Chapter 3: Healthy Tips 14

A FEW TIPS: 14
B12 Supplements: 14
Iron Supplements: 15
Consume Abundant Protein In Your Diet: 16
Making A Change Is Not That Easy: 16
Be Cautious With What You Buy: 17
NUTRITIONAL STATUS OF VEGAN DIET: 18

Chapter 4: Benefitsof Vegan Diet 20

HEALTH BENEFITS OF THE VEGAN DIET: 20
BENEFITS OF A HEALTHIER BODY WITH THE VEGAN DIET: 24

Chapter 5: Drawbacks Of Vegan Diet 28

DRAWBACKS OF THE VEGAN DIET: 28
SUMMARY: 31

Chapter 6:Vegan Diet Plan 33

VEGAN DIET PLAN: 34
Breakfast: *34*
Lunch: *35*
Dinner: *36*
Snacks: *37*

Chapter 7: Vegan Slow Cooker 38

VEGAN SLOW COOKER RECIPES: 39
VEGAN CHOCOLATE PUDDING: 39

Chapter 8:Vegan Body Building 42

Protein Shakes: *43*

Chapter 9: A Few Recommendations And Tips.................. 44

Conclusion: 46

Part 2 49

Introduction 50

Chapter 1 - Protein.. 56

Chapter 2 – 15 Tantalizing Breakfast Recipes.................... 63

Strawberry Oatmeal Breakfast Smoothie.......................... 63

Vegan Jelly Filled Muffins 64

3. Vegan Breakfast Bowl 66

4. Pancakes 67

5. Banana And Berry Smoothie 69

Pumpkin Bread 70

7. Tofu 'Eggs' 72

8. Chorizo" Breakfast Tacos 73

9. Banana And Blueberry Bars 76

10. Breakfast Burrito 78

11. Oat Cookies 82

12. Vegan Cheese Omelet 84

13. Pumpkin Oatmeal Recipe 85

14. Basic Scrambled Tofu 86

15. Vegan Granola Bars 88

Chapter 3 – 16 Delicious Lunch Recipes 91

2. Parsnip Pear Soup 93

3. Crab Cakes 94

4. Mushroom, Corn, And Black Bean Farro 97

5. Kale Quinoa Salad With Red Grapes 99

6. White Bean Salad With Olives And Arugula 101

7. Veggie And Hummus Sandwich 102

8. Soy-Lime Tofu & Rice Bento Lunch 103

10. Quinoa Salad With Creamy Avocado Dressing 107

11. Coconut Curry Lentil Soup 109

12. Easy Lemon Lentil Soup 111

13. Refreshing Quinoa Salad With Mango, Cucumber, Avocado & Black Beans 112

14. Grilled Mediterranean Vegetables On White Bean Mash 113

15. Cauliflower And Lentil Coconut Curry 115

16. Healthy Vegan Quinoa Chili 117

Chapter 4 – 10 Delightful Dinner Recipes 120

2. Sweet Potato & Black Bean Veggie Burgers 122

3. Chopped Kale Salad With Edamame, Carrot And Avocado 125

4. Spicy Roasted Ratatouille With Spaghetti 127

5. Butternut Squash Chipotle Chili With Avocado 130

6. Creamy Roasted Brussels Sprout And Quinoa Gratin ... 133

7. Three Bean Chili With Spring Pesto 135

8. Swiss Chard With Chickpeas And Couscous 137

9. Linguine With Caper And Green Olive Sauce 138

10. Baked Macaroni And Cheese 139

Chapter 5 – 10 Revitalizing Meal Plans 143

Breakfast 144

Conclusion 147

About The Author 150

Part 1

INTRODUCTION

Now veganism is a very broad term. It basically involves the abstaining of animal products. If restricted to the diet, such people are known as dietary vegans. If it involves boycotting of all animal related goods for example bags, shoes, for entertainment purposes etc, such people are called ethical vegans. Now this abstaining of animal related goods or products may be due to different reasons. For some, it is a matter of religion or culture. This can be explained by its historical background which dates back to the time when it was first practiced in India and Ancient Greece. For example the Hindu culture in India considers cows to be holy. Hence, it is a sin for them to kill animals and consume their meat. Those who practice Hinduism truly will also be true vegans.

The other aspect here is that some people may switch to a vegan diet as it offers different benefits mainly health related. They will be discussed in detail later in this book. It must be noted here that vegans and vegetarians are not the same. The difference is that vegans do not consume animal related products at all like meat, eggs, dairy products etc. However, vegetarians only abstain from meat. Ethical vegans go a step further and do not use anything related to animals as they believe it is against the ethics to kill animals or to make them suffer. So what do vegans eat? Their diet basically contains grains, legumes, vegetables, fruits, nuts etc. Soy is also another staple diet for vegans as it is rich in proteins. Then there are the environmental vegans who abstain from animal related products as they believe it causes environmental destruction in different ways. This will be explained in more detail in the following chapters.

However, our emphasis in this book will be on vegan diet. The purpose is to guide you towards dietary veganism whether you are merely interested to learn more about it or you want to switch to a vegan diet. No matter what your reason is, this is a complete guide book which will lead you step by step towards understanding what the vegan diet really is, the benefits it has to offer and how to successfully switch to it if that is what you are looking for. Information will be given on the different types of vegans and how each of them differs. In addition,we will provide you with the best alternatives to make your diet complete and fulfilling despite the restrictions of the vegan diet. This is essential to keep your diet balanced so that you receive all the important nutrients that you need to stay healthy.

CHAPTER 1:GETTING STARTED

What is Veganism?

Veganism is

the abstaining of all animal products such that vegans (the people who practice veganism) do not consume animal meat, fish, poultry etc. In addition, they abstain from all sorts of animal products like eggs, dairy products, even honey and in some cases all kinds of products manufactured from animals for example bags, shoes, clothes, make up etc.

What is the difference between vegetarians and vegans?

Vegetarians abstain from animal meat including that of poultry, seafood etc. However they do not abstain from any animal products.

Vegans abstain from animal meat of all sorts as well as eggs, dairy products and other products manufactured from animals.

What are the different types of veganism?

1. Health veganism
2. Environmental veganism
3. Ethical veganism
4. Others

Health veganism:

Due to certain health benefits associated with the vegan diet, some people exclude meat and animal products from their diets to minimize the harmful effects that it imposes on their bodies. The health benefits will be discussed in detail in the proceeding chapters.

Environmental veganism:

This class of people focuses on conserving the environment and hence do not favor any practices that can cause a threat to the environment such as hunting, fishing

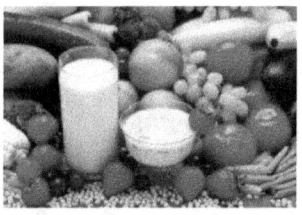

etc. It also focuses on the fact that farming of animals limits the land resources and hence it should not be favored.

Ethical veganism:

It is argued by this particular group that animals should not be killed for food, entertainment etc. This is because they possess rights just like humans do. They believe that animal life must not be devalued just because they belong to a different species. Hence, such people not only exclude animal meat, eggs, dairy products and honey from their diets but do not use anything associated with animals. For example animal skin clothes, shoes, make up tested or derived from animals etc.

Others:

Now this includes cultural veganism. In some religions/cultures, animals are considered holy creatures. Hence, their meat or their products are not consumed for it is sinful for them, for example Hindus.

The other class is temporary but may be included here. It includes the class of people that are not economically stable. In fact, such people strive to fulfill their basic resources and all they can afford is grains and legumes.

CHAPTER 2: IMPORTANT QUESTIONS

What does the Vegan diet include?

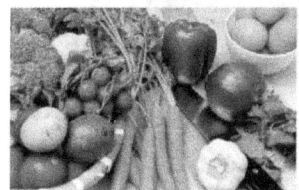

Vegan diet includes all vegetables, fruits, grains, legumes, beans etc. In addition there is soy milk which opens up a lot of options for you since you do not consume dairy milk. There is also tofu which is basically curd that is made from mashed soybeans. It is typically used in vegan cooking.

What does the Vegan diet exclude?

Vegan diet excludes all sorts of animal meat be it of cows, goats, chicken, turkey, duck, seafood etc. In addition, it also

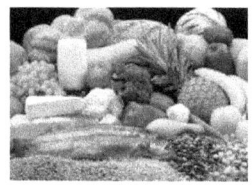

excludes animal products such as eggs, dairy products, honey etc.

How do you substitute for dairy products?

This question is typically concerning for the majority as they find it difficult to change their lifestyle so drastically. Many people who are tea or coffee drinkers are concerned how to lead their lives without it. One possible alternative is to develop the taste of tea or coffee without milk. You may switch to green tea instead as well.

However, if you just cannot stay away from milk or other dairy products, there are a few alternatives for you. These days, there is an availability of non dairy products which can be used as a substitution for milk such as soymilk, almond milk, rice milk.

In addition, you may consume vegan margarine which is non dairy. There are also non dairy soy cheese, non dairy cheese sauces, non dairy sour cream, non dairy ice creams etc. Hence, if you explore your options, you will find a lot of substitutes which can make this switching to the vegan diet easier for you. The best part is that for the most part, these are now readily available and also cheap. Also, they are a lot healthier than dairy milk considering their fat and cholesterol content. Soy milk also has the advantage of being high in protein.

The non dairy substitutes are an excellent alternative for those who are lactose intolerant. Also, they have less fat and cholesterol and hence you may be able to control your cholesterol as well as your weight better. You can use these non dairy products to make cookies, cakes, pastas etc. Hence, all you need to do is make a little more effort for your health in order to eat whatever you like.

Are there any substitutes for eggs

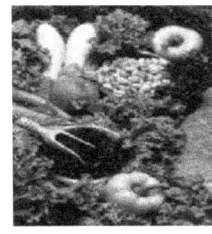

suitable for my Vegan diet?

Yes!

You can use different substitutes if you want to exclude eggs from your diet due to egg allergies or if you are switching to a vegan diet.

One of them is known as the Ener-G. This can be used as an alternative to eggs.

However, they do not have much flavor so they are better suited to baked foods where you may require eggs for example cakes, cookies etc.

Tofu is another substitute for eggs which is very much suitable for vegans. We also have another mixture that we can use as a substitute to eggs in baking. This is by combining bananas and apple sauce. Surprisingly, it works like eggs do in baking stuff like cupcakes, cookies etc.

Therefore, you can use different alternatives for eggs conveniently which are also healthy such that they are low in cholesterol.

CHAPTER 3: HEALTHY TIPS

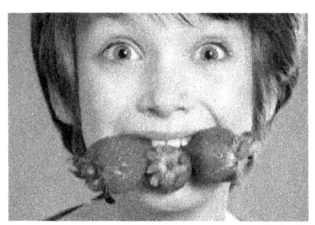

Now you may be switching to vegan because of your belief in animal rights and hence you may not believe in slaughtering them for food, entertainment etc. You might be switching to it because you want to conserve the environment. On the other hand, you may be switching to it because of its various health benefits. No matter what your reason is, you need to know a few important aspects before you switch to a vegan diet. We have summarized them for you below.

A FEW TIPS:

B12 supplements:

Animal food contains B12 naturally. By going vegan, you may make your body deficient of this vitamin B12. Hence, you must take vitamin B12 supplements or consume food that contains more of this vitamin to prevent your body from its deficiency. Now you need to know why it is important for you in the first place. Vitamin B12 is essential in the normal functioning of the body such that it is needed by your body's blood cells and nerve bundles to make DNA. If this function fails, it can result in your nerve functions to be impaired. In addition, it will make you tired and weak; you may not feel hungry and lose weight unnaturally. Constipation is very common in such cases too. In extreme cases, you may feel depressed very often.

Iron supplements:

Now iron deficiency can cause you to become dizzy, have headaches, feel weak and fatigued etc. Vegan diet does contain iron but it is the non-heme kind. On the contrary, animal diet contains more iron of the form, heme. The advantage of heme is that it easily absorbed by the body as compared to non-heme. Hence, your body may become deficient of iron if you are switching to vegan. For this purpose, you must either take iron supplements or consume green vegetables abundantly, legumes, sunflower seeds etc to help in the absorption of iron in your body to prevent its deficiency.

Consume abundant protein in your diet:

Animal meat and eggs are an abundant source of proteins. If you are switching to vegan, you may need to ensure that you increase your protein intake from other foods for example beans, soy etc.

Making a change is not that easy:

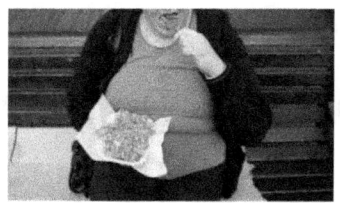

It is certainly not easy making any change overnight and this case is no different. Hence, you must be determined to switch to it willingly. Also, it is a good idea to take things step by step. You may want to add more vegetables, fruits etc in your diet while decreasing the intake of animal meat and related products successively over a period of time. This is a better idea instead of starting the vegan diet and giving up in frustration.

Be cautious with what you buy:

Many foods contain animal products even if they do not seem like it. Hence, you must be cautious while buying processed foods etc. Checking labels and their ingredients is a good idea in order to stick to your vegan diet.

Nutritional status of Vegan diet:

- Vegan diet is rich in **calcium** if you consume lots of green vegetables, tofu etc. You may not need take any additional supplements in most cases if your diet is sufficient.
- **Vitamin D** is not found in the vegan diet. However, that can be compensated by exposure to sunlight. You may want to spend some time in the sun letting it fall on your exposed skin to stimulate the production of Vitamin D. Two to three times a week is recommended for at least fifteen minutes during the day. In addition, you can supplement Vitamin D in your diet by consuming vitamin D-fortified soy milk or rice milk.
- Vegan diet is typically low in **fats and cholesterol**. However, this is to your advantage as you do not need high levels of either of these in your body. It

prevents many diseases which will be discussed in the next chapter in detail.

- **Zinc** is found in abundance in legumes, grains, nuts etc. Hence, vegan diets provide you with this advantage. Zinc is essential to your body in different ways. It helps build your immune system and is also needed to make proteins, DNA and other genetic material in your body.
- **Iron**is found in green leafy vegetables, beans etc. However, vegan diet mostly contains the non-heme kind of iron which is not readily absorbed by the body. Hence iron supplements may need to be taken.
- **Vitamin B12** is mostly absent from vegan diets. Hence, you may need to supplement your body by taking these vitamins additionally.

CHAPTER 4: BENEFITS OF VEGAN DIET

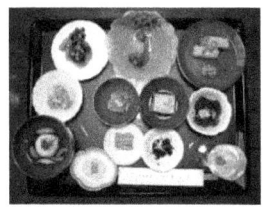

Switching to vegan has many health benefits which is precisely one of the reasons why some people choose to bring about this change in their lives. It is healthier in most cases and prevents against many diseases. We will discuss the health benefits in detail in this chapter so that you can have a comprehensive outlook of it.

Health Benefits of the Vegan diet:

- Switching to a vegan diet automatically cuts down the fats in your diet. Hence, it makes weight loss easier for those who intend on getting slimmer. For others, it is a healthy way to keep in

shape. A diet with low fats reduces the risk of cardiovascular diseases.
- A vegan diet is rich in fiber. This improves your peristaltic movements and helps against constipation. Thus, it is a good way of regulating your digestive system. In addition, it fights against colon cancer.
- Calcium is important in the diet. Its absorption is helped by magnesium. Magnesium is found abundantly in your vegan diet in the form of green vegetables, nuts etc. Hence, it helps aid the absorption of calcium in your body. In addition, it helps prevent osteoporosis by maintaining a balance of minerals in the body.
- Potassium is found in high levels in this diet. Potassium is important in the acid-base balance of your body. It reduces the acidity and helps eliminate the toxins in your body via the kidneys. This is also helpful in reducing the risk of

cardiovascular diseases and certain cancers.
- Fruits and vegetables are an excellent source of Vitamin C, especially citrus fruits. This promotes healing and helps against bleeding gums. In addition, it is also an antioxidant which helps prevent different cancers and also helps against the damage of cells in your body.
- Vitamin E is good for your body in so many ways such as the skin, eyes, brain etc. Green vegetables and nuts provide you with sufficient Vitamin E.
- Problems of uric acid and gout are common in many individuals. This is due to a high intake of protein in the diet which is mainly taken from animal meat. Vegetables, nuts, beans etc have protein in a balanced form such that it fulfills your body requirements and ensures that it is not taken in excess. Hence, it helps prevent diseases resulting from high protein intake.

- Phytochemicals are substances specifically found in plants. Hence, vegan diet provides you with phytochemicals in your body. These are helpful in preventing cancers.
- Animal meat is rich in cholesterol. By switching to vegan, the cholesterol levels are much lower in your bodies and hence help against any heart diseases.
- Grains are a major part of the vegan diet. They offer you the advantage of keeping your blood pressure low and hence preventing hypertension due to high blood pressure.
- Vegan diet helps prevent Type 2 diabetes.
- Certain cancers are prevented by the vegan diet. These include colon cancer due to the high consumption of fiber in the diet, prostate cancer as well as breast cancer which is more common in women who consume more animal meat.

- As stated before, vegan diet is rich in vitamin E which is beneficial for you in different ways such as the eyes. It helps prevent cataract due to the presence of antioxidants in your body.
- A vegan diet helps improve the symptoms of rheumatoid arthritis. This is because of the exclusion of dairy products from the diet which is thought to be linked with the worsening of the symptoms of arthritis.

Hence, we have discussed some of the most important health benefits linked with the vegan diet and the diseases it is capable of preventing. It also has other benefits which can help your body appear healthier. They are enumerated as below.

Benefits of a healthier body with the vegan diet:

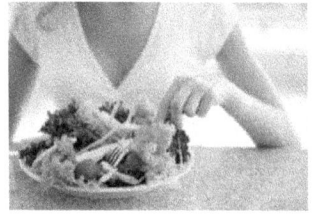

Stay in shape now with a balanced consumption of fats in your diet. It not only helps against weight loss but also helps you stay in a healthy shape.
- Enjoy healthy and clear skin with this diet. It has the right amount of antioxidants, zinc, Vitamin E etc.
- The hair is nourished from within by the vitamins and minerals consumed in this diet. Hence, it appears healthier and stronger.
- Nails, like hair are nourished by vitamins and minerals consumed in the vegan diet.
- Body odor is associated with animal meats and dairy products. Hence, the vegan diet allows you to eliminate or lessen your body odor.
- Bad breath is also associated with the consumption of animal meats and dairy products. Hence, you may help decrease that by going vegan.
- Interestingly, vegans are associated with fewer migraines. Hence, if you are an individual who suffers from chronic

migraine, you might want to switch to veganism.

- Many allergies are associated with meat, dairy products and eggs. Hence, vegans may have lesser allergies or if you are allergic to either of these foods, you may experience relief of your allergic symptoms.

Therefore, you have seen the various health benefits in terms of the different diseases you can prevent as well as the outward effect on your bodies by going vegan. It can correctly be said that veganism is a healthy form of eating which makes your body feel healthy from within, or be healthy inside out.

Hence, some people switch to a vegan diet simply to lead a healthier lifestyle and stay away from unhealthy or processed foods which can cause harm to your body in different ways such as heart diseases, cancers etc. For some individuals, the reason may be as simple as weight loss.

Regardless, switching to veganism has immense benefits and may not be a bad option if you want to switch to a healthy form of eating.

CHAPTER 5: DRAWBACKS OF VEGAN DIET

We have discussed veganism in detail by now. The previous chapter was dedicated to the benefits of the vegan diet. However, there may be a few drawbacks of the vegan diet as well. There is argument that there is no correct way or there is no one way of eating. It differs from person to person and their circumstances. This might be true to some extent. Hence, we will now discuss a different aspect of veganism and its drawbacks.

Drawbacks of the Vegan diet:

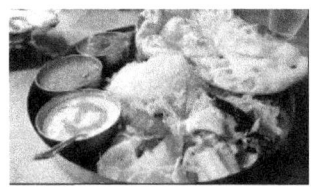

Your body needs different nutrients to function efficiently. The ideal way of eating is to consume a balanced diet. Animals and plants contain different type of nutrients. Collectively, you are able to consume the different nutrients that your body needs as some nutrients are absent in plants and vice versa.

An example is of vitamin B12 which was discussed in the previous chapter as well. It is important for the body cells, to make DNA and for the efficient functioning of the brain. However, it is absent in plants. Hence, an individual who consumes a vegan diet will be deficient of this vitamin. He/she will experience symptoms of tiredness, weakness, lethargy etc. Although, supplements may be taken, it cannot replace the natural form of nutrients.

There are other examples as well for example animals contain creatine which is important for the proper functioning of the brain and muscles. In vegans, it is absent and hence may create different problems.

- Now it is important to know that a study must be conducted with consistent results for it to be successful. In the case of vegan diet, there is no known study that suggests its authenticity in it being better than other diets. It may work better for some people while on the other hand, other diets are better for others. This in a way concludes that there can be no fixed diet for everyone. There are variations in every individual and hence it is a matter of one's personal preference and their body responses.

- While it may be true about the harmful effects of animal meat, eggs etc, it cannot be denied that they have immense benefits for the body too. Hence, it may be argued that removing them completely from the diet is not a wise decision.

In fact, removing animal meat and products from the diet may result in your body getting deficient of various minerals and vitamins. Hence, you may need to be extra cautious about that as well as need to take artificial diet supplements.

If you must make a change, you may be decide to be careful about the animal meat that you buy such that it is grass fed and is not brought up unnaturally in any form. This way, you can avoid the processed meat and the chemicals associated with it that may prove harmful to your body. Similarly, you may consume **Omega 3 rich eggs and fresh dairy milk instead of consuming the processed milk which has preservatives.**

Summary:

Now the purpose to give the drawbacks here was that you must have the complete knowledge on the vegan diet including its advantages and disadvantages. The decision is entirely up to you. However, what was emphasized in this chapter was that there is no single way you must eat. Every person varies according to their health, genetics, preference, circumstances, lifestyle etc.

You cannot just base your diet on one factor which is the reason why some people respond well to certain diets and others do not. There is no scientific evidence to prove that vegan diets are better than other diets though some people have shown remarkable improvement in their health as well as standard of living by switching to vegan.

Another important aspect that was discussed indicated that animal diet is very nutritious and has several benefits to the body. By switching to vegan, you deprive your body of that nutrition and make it deficient in some important minerals and vitamins that need to be supplemented in order for your body to function normally.

CHAPTER 6: VEGAN DIET PLAN

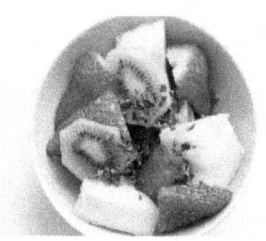

Now meals are an important part of the day for most of us. Switching to a vegan diet might have you concerned over how you will plan your meals and how to start it. You need not worry as we will provide you with a complete vegan diet plan.

The essential part is for you to get started. We will provide you with a vegan diet guide in the form of a vegan cookbook which will include a few bonus recipes for you to get started. Once you start reading ahead, you will see that vegan cooking is not so difficult after all. In fact, you can experiment to make delicious food. In addition, it is not so boring to be a vegan. Like it was discussed in the first chapter, there are various alternatives available to you instead of dairy products, eggs etc. You may need to develop a taste for them but you will not be missing out on much that way.

Vegan diet plan:

Vegan diet plans like discussed before allow you to lose your weight by consuming healthy foods while cutting down on the fats in your diet. The best part is that you need not starve yourself. You may consume three meals a day while at the same time use this diet plan for effective weight loss.

Bonus recipes/ideas have been included for each meal to give you a kick start.

Breakfast:

Cereal with milk suitable for vegans. You may choose between soy milk, almond milk, rice milk etc. For the cereal, you may choose any that is suitable for vegans. You must read the labels carefully and read into the ingredients. Oatmeal may also be taken.

Fruits are an excellent source of energy and are antioxidants. These can be added to the breakfast to make it into a fulfilling meal for example berries, bananas etc.

- You may take soy yoghurt and add granola to it. In addition, you can add fruits to complete your meal.
- A fruit smoothie makes a wonderful breakfast. It is fulfilling and delicious. Add in berries or your favorite fruits along with milk suitable for vegans. This can be soy milk, almond milk, rice milk etc.
- You miss eggs? Do not worry for you have tofu. Make a scrambled tofu breakfast as an alternative to eggs. You may add spices and vegetables according to your taste.

Lunch:

- Salads make an excellent lunch. They are healthy and fulfilling and not difficult to make. The only precaution you need here is that you must read labels of dressings that you use carefully. Apart from that, you may toss in all your favorite vegetables and add some delicious dressing for flavor and dig in.
- Sandwiches can be made for lunch. You may add tomatoes, lettuce, tofu etc depending on your taste and what you want to eat. These are again easy to make and healthy as well.
- Soups are delicious and fulfilling. You can make a variety of soups depending on your taste. Examples are leak and carrot ginger soup, potato leak soup etc.

Dinner:

- For dinner, you can make yourself some lasagna. All you need is lasagna strips, non dairy cheese, green vegetables etc depending on what filling you want to have. Pizza is also a viable option if you

ensure that the dough is vegan suitable and the cheese you buy is non dairy.
- You can make yourself some pasta using vegetables only. For flavor, you may add different spices.
- Beans are perfectly suitable for your vegan diet and also very healthy. You may choose to have these as a side to your main course.
- Then again, you can make soups, salads and sandwiches as per the requirement of vegans.

Snacks:

- Fruits are an excellent snack. A banana, apple, berries etc would do the trick for you.
- A fruit smoothie like the one that was recommended for breakfast is a good snack and also replenishes your energy.
- Oven baked tortilla chips with salsa makes a delicious snack.

CHAPTER 7: VEGAN SLOW COOKER

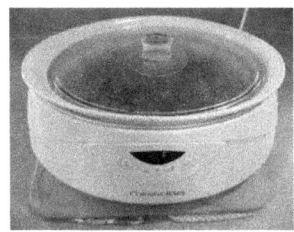

We have discussed your basic vegan diet plan and guided you towards it. As discussed in the previous chapter, we gave you a few basic ideas and recipes to get you started on your vegan diet. Another aspect we will discuss here is how to cook a vegan diet with a slow cooker.

This has been added as some people like cooking on a slow cooker. This is due to a variety of reasons. They are cheaper to buy, more energy efficient and hence economical to use. Some people are used to cooking on a slow cooker. Soups, stews, vegan casseroles etc may be made using it. Hence, we will discuss how to cook a vegan diet using it. One bonus recipe has been added in this chapter.

So basically, we are going to guide you to use a slow cooker to make a vegan diet. This is unusual as meats are basically cooked on slow cookers as in stews.

Vegan slow cooker recipes:

There are countless vegan foods you can make on a slow cooker from appetizers to the main courses and desserts. As a bonus, we have added a recipe for you.

Vegan chocolate pudding:

(Made in a slow cooker)

Ingredients:
- All purpose flour: 1 cup
- Sugar: ½ cup
- Cocoa powder: 2tbsp and ¼ cup
- Baking powder: 2tsp

- Salt: ½ tsp
- Soymilk: ½ cup
- Vegetable oil: 2 tbsp
- Vanilla: 1 tsp
- Brown sugar: ¾ cup
- Hot water: 1 ½ cup

Directions:

- Take a large bowl and mix in the flour, sugar, 2 tbspcocoa powder, baking powder and salt.
- Add oil, soy milk and vanilla in the mixture.
- Use a cooking spray to spray inside the crock pot before pouring in the batter.
- Use the remaining ¼ cup of cocoa powder and brown sugar and mix until smooth. Pour this over the batter then.
- Pour hot water inside the crock pot without stirring.
- Cook in the crock pot for 2 hours. Check with a toothpick to ensure it has been cooked properly. If toothpick comes out clean, you may stop cooking.

- Take off the lid and let it stand for half an hour.
- Take out the cake in your desired dishes and garnish.
- You may use soy whipped cream or chocolate sauce.

CHAPTER 8: VEGAN BODY BUILDING

We shall talk on another aspect here, vegan body building. This is also to clear the misconception that you cannot build up your body without animal diet which contains essential amino acids. The fact is that you can build your body and have strong muscles with a vegan diet.

There are two important things that you must do with a vegan diet. They are:

Training/ exercises

Protein shakes

Training:

It is very important to have a proper training routine to build up your muscles. You may work out in different ways such as squats, bench presses, dips, chin ups etc.

It is also important to carry out a proper routine such that you work out for a specific time period every day or a few days in a week.

Protein shakes:

Your muscle mass requires proteins. A vegan diet provides you with ample proteins in your diet. However, you will need protein shakes with that extra muscle building.

To make your own, buy any protein powder that you like from your local markets. Mix in 3 tbsp with 8oz of almond milk and 8oz of soy milk. You can also add in fresh fruits to give a smoothie effect or to enhance the taste. It also makes it extra nutritious and refreshing. It is preferable that you take your protein shake after your work out.

CHAPTER 9: A FEW RECOMMENDATIONS AND TIPS

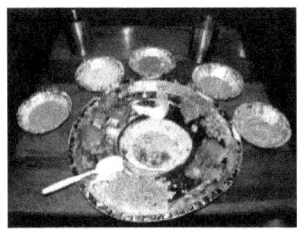

- Switching to a vegan diet is not hard if you are motivated towards it owing to your own personal reasons. However, you will need to pay more attention to the labels while buying different foods to ensure that they are suitable for you.
- Different alternatives are available in the market for the exclusions in the vegan diet. Hence, you may make full use of these to cook up food that you love. Remember, you can always experiment according to your taste.

This is also a weight loss diet but you need not worry about consuming too much when it comes to fruits, vegetables, grains and beans. This is because of their fat content which is very low.

Cereal, bread etc are all acceptable but you must ensure that the ingredients are friendly towards your diet. It is better to avoid, sugar, corn syrup and other chemical preservatives.

- Fruits are excellent for salads, snacks etc. However, it is better to consume the ones with no extra sugar.
- You can consume grains with no worries of consuming too much. However, it would just be ideal if you choose the grains with fiber in them for extra health benefits.

CONCLUSION:

This book was developed as a beginners guide to the vegan diet. It was meant to equip you with all the necessary knowledge on what the vegan diet really is, its benefits and drawbacks, how it is different from the vegetarian diet, the different types of veganism and their details etc. It has numerous health benefits which were discussed in detail. In addition, it provided you with essential ideas that you can use to get started on your vegan diet with a complete vegan diet plan to guide you properly. Whether you are just a keen reader interested to gain knowledge or looking for a healthy form of diet/ lifestyle, this book was meant for you as it is comprehensive and helpful.

The vegan diet has a few dietary modifications. Some people find these very concerning and a lot of stress was given on the alternatives present to the exclusions of the vegan diet to make you aware of the different alternatives present. In addition, different ideas were presented to you respectively to cook up a healthy and fulfilling meal for breakfast, lunch, dinner as well as snacking. A few bonus recipes were added to give you a start as well.

The book was compiled in a way to make it easy to read with bullet points, headings and subheadings. In addition, a few summaries and tips were added to facilitate your learning and grasp on the topic. In general, it is stated that diets may differ for every individual depending on their genetics, circumstances, lifestyle etc. The vegan diet is one form of diet that you may switch to. It offers you a chance to eat healthy and cut down on junk food, foods high in cholesterol, fat etc. Therefore, it plays an important part in weight loss. You may follow the diet without starving yourself and still maintain a good shape.

A chapter was also added on body building using vegan diet to assure you that with the right training and supplements, you can make your muscles stronger and also build up your body. Hence, it leaves your body strong, healthy and energized. Therefore, effort was made to cover every aspect of the topic to answer any general questions that may arise commonly in your minds. The nutritional status of the vegan diet was also discussed in detail to indicate which vitamins and minerals it provides you and which it does not. The problems or were also discussed along with their solutions on how to supplement for the deficiencies of the vegan diet.

Overall, we hope this book was beneficial for you as a beginner. We hope you have gained enough knowledge now to understand the concept of veganism and the vegan diet. We also hope that you can now benefit yourself directly by following this vegan diet and prevent yourself and your loved ones against a variety of diseases.

Part 2

Introduction

The decision to adopt a vegan lifestyle is not one which should be taken lightly, being a vegan means refraining from eating any animal product. It can be both challenging and extremely rewarding; changing from eating meat can be difficult as you may not be able to see how you can enjoy food as much as you currently do. In fact, there is an abundance of different food sources available which will not only replace meat, but will actually taste better and potentially offer health benefits. Even if you are fully prepared for the change in your lifestyle and, in particular, eating habits, you may experience some negative reactions from friends, family and colleagues who do not understand the principles and many will be afraid to prepare you food in the future!

The main reason for choosing a vegan lifestyle is because you believe that all living beings have a right to life and freedom; this means you are unwilling to eat any animal or animal related product. The belief will stretch to all areas of life, particularly beauty products; some of which are still tested on animals.

The vegan lifestyle is also an excellent way to show that you care for the environment; recycling is becoming common place and many people are looking to reduce their own carbon footprint. Becoming vegan will ensure you minimize your effect on the environment.

Of course, many people may argue that eating animals is the best way of controlling the animal population; however, it is often the case that vast amounts of land are used to grow crops simply to feed the animals. This land could be used to grow food for humans and significantly less land would be required!

Veganism is becoming a more popular choice and this does make it easier to switch eating habits, more products are available in the supermarkets than ever before.

One of the biggest issues which have always faced those wishing to pursue a life of veganism is protein. Meat is an excellent source of protein and is known as a 'complete protein'. In essence this is any protein which contains the nine essential amino acids. Protein is made up of amino acids and there are twenty different ones which are vital for the general health of the body, of these twenty there are nine which the body is not able to produce by itself. These nine are known as the essential amino acids as they are required by your body but you are unable to produce them yourself; they must be consumed. Thankfully meat is not the only source of these proteins! Eggs and diary are also an excellent source of complete protein; unfortunately these are also not an option for the committed vegan. This is exactly why many people state that the vegan diet is not healthy.

There are actually an abundance of other foods which do contain these essential amino acids; it is actually very easy to consume all of the necessary nutrients in one day providing you understand which food sources are rich in these essential nutrients. It is perhaps more important to ensure you eat a balanced diet, after all, the average man only requires sixty three grams of protein a day, whilst the average female needs fifty two grams per day, this roughly equates to one calorie of every ten consumed needing to be protein based. A varied plant based diet will provide all the protein that you require and avoid any health issues, such as kidney disease or osteoporosis which have been linked to excessive protein consumption.

This book will provide you with information regarding the best sources of protein; these food sources can be added to any meal to increase your protein intake. There is also an example of a menu plan for a day and fifty one recipes, providing breakfast, lunch and dinner suggestions.

Chapter 1 - Protein

As mentioned, protein is essential to the human body; the following food types are all rich in protein and are acceptable to those living a vegan lifestyle:

- Quinoa – This looks very similar to couscous but is much more nutritious. It is an excellent replacement for rice and is full of fiber, iron and magnesium. It has eight grams of protein per serving.
- Buckwheat – This is actually a type of rhubarb and not wheat as its name suggests. It is commonly ground into flour and can then be used in a variety of recipes. It contains six grams of protein per serving and has been shown to improve your circulation as

well as lower cholesterol and possibly blood sugar levels.

- Hempseed – This is a natural source of essential fatty acids and magnesium, zinc, iron and calcium; as well as having ten grams of protein per serving.
- Chia – These seeds can be combined with water to make a gel like substance which has proved to be excellent for making puddings. They are extremely high in iron, zinc, calcium and antioxidants and also contain omega 3 fatty acids, fiber and four grams of protein per serving.
- Soy – This is one of the original food sources for vegans, also known as tofu. The firmer the tofu the better the protein content. Tempeh and Natto

both have fifteen grams per serving whilst tofu has ten grams.

- Quorn – This product is grown in vats and was originally developed to assist with global food shortage issues. It is manufactured into a meat substitute and is a source of complete protein. It is important to be careful when selecting Quorn products – some products use egg whites and are not vegan friendly. It has thirteen grams of protein per serving.
- Rice and Beans - Rice is known to be high in methionine and low in lysine whilst beans are the opposite. Put the two together in a meal and you will have a complete source of protein! The

average serving will contain seven grams of protein.

- Ezekiel Bread – This bread was referred to in the bible and is made from wheat, barley, beans, lentils, millet and spelt. It contains eight grams of protein per two slice serving.
- Seitan – This is also known as wheat gluten and is an excellent as a meat substitute; although obviously of little use to those who are intolerant of gluten. The seitan should be cooked in a soy sauce to ensure all the essential amino acids are present. It will then contain twenty one grams of protein per serving.
- Hummus and Pita – This is another combination which fits perfectly

together; the high lysine content in the hummus complements the pita to give seven grams of protein per serving.

There are, of course, many other food sources of protein and they can all be mixed and matched to ensure you reach the necessary amount of protein each day. Below is an example of a menu for a day, this will provide more protein than you need:

Breakfast: Oatmeal, soy milk and a medium bagel

Lunch: Whole wheat bread and baked beans

Dinner: Firm tofu, broccoli, almonds and brown rice

Snack: Crackers and peanut butter

Total protein content from the above food would be seventy seven grams.

Protein can be found in varying degrees in most vegetables, grains, beans, nuts and seeds. A balanced diet will ensure you receive enough protein daily.

There are also several protein powders on the market which are designed to supplement the vegan lifestyle.

Here are a few:

Pea Protein

Soy Protein Isolate

Brown Rice

Hemp Protein

Multi-Blend Protein

Generally Vegan protein powders will vary from 10g to 20g protein per serving.

These supplements can be used to ensure you are consuming a balance, nutritious diet or they can be used to assist with building and repairing muscles. These supplements can offer valuable support but should not be taken as a replacement for a meal; there are many other nutrients which are present in your food and all are just as important for your health.

Chapter 2 – 15 Tantalizing Breakfast Recipes

Breakfast is the most important meal of the day. It fires up your metabolism at the start of each day and provides you with energy to keep you going all day long. The following recipes are all excellent ways to start the day and keep your hunger at bay all morning.

Strawberry Oatmeal Breakfast Smoothie

Ingredients

- 1 cup soy milk
- ½ cup rolled oats
- 1 banana - sliced
- 14 frozen strawberries
- ½ tsp vanilla extract
  - 1 ½ tsp white sugar

Instructions

1. Combine the soy milk, oats, banana and strawberries in a blender.

2. Add the vanilla, and sugar, if desired and blend again until smooth.
3. Pour into a glass and enjoy!

Vegan Jelly Filled Muffins

Ingredients

- 1 ½ cups all purpose flour
- ¾ tsp baking powder
- ½ tsp baking soda
- ½ tsp ground nutmeg
- salt
- 1 cup plain rice/soy milk
- 1 tsp cider vinegar
- 2 tbsp cornstarch
- ¾ cup sugar
- ½ cup vegetable oil
- 2 tsp vanilla extract
- ½ cup raspberry, strawberry or grape jam

Instructions

1. Line a muffin pan and pre-heat the oven to 350 F.

2. Mix the flour, baking powder, baking soda, nutmeg and salt in a mixing bowl. Make a well in the centre of the bowl and leave to one side for a moment.

   Next whisk together the soy/rice milk, vinegar and cornstarch until all ingredients have dissolved. Pour this liquid mix into the well in the flour mixture. Then add the sugar, oil and vanilla and stir. Ideally you should stir with a rubber spatula; there will be a few lumps.
4. Fill each muffin well to approximately three quarters full. Create a small indentation in the batter with a spoon by spreading the mixture slightly from the middle outward. Place one teaspoon of jam in the indentation.
5. Cook in the preheated oven until the tops of the muffins are firm, this should be approximately twenty to twenty five minutes. The muffins should then be allowed to cool for five minutes on a wire rack before they are consumed.

3. Vegan Breakfast Bowl

Ingredients

- ½ lb. extra-firm tofu – this will need to be drained and cut into cubes
- Olive oil
- 1 tbsp. soy sauce
- Pinch of basil
- Pinch of oregano
- 1 cup cooked brown rice
- 1 tbsp miso paste
- ½ bunch broccoli – to be cut into florets and then steamed
- ½ cooked sweet potato - diced
- 1 carrot - shredded
- 1 tsp sauerkraut
- 1 tsp pickled ginger – if required

Instructions

1. Mix the tofu, olive oil, soy sauce, basil, and oregano together and heat until the tofu is a golden brown.

2. Next combine the cooked brown rice and miso paste, add the tofu mixture, broccoli,

sweet potato, carrot, sauerkraut, and, if required, the pickled ginger.

3. Serve immediately and enjoy the variety of flavors.

4. Pancakes

Ingredients

- 1 cup all-purpose flour
- 1 tbsp sugar
- 2 tbsp baking powder
- Pinch of salt
- 1 cup soy milk
- 1 scoop of a Vegan protein powder
- 2 tbsp vegetable oil
- Your choice of topping

Instructions

1. Place the flour, sugar, protein powder, baking powder, and salt in a bowl and mix together. Then add the soy milk and oil before mixing further until the batter is smooth. An electric whisk can make this job easier!

2. To make a pancake pour approximately half a cup of the batter onto a hot griddle – making sure it is oiled first. It should take around two minutes to cook one side of the pancake; you will know it is done as you will see bubbles on the top surface of the pancake. Turn the pancake over and cook the second side.

3. It is a good idea to have the oven on a low heat whilst making the pancakes. As each one is ready you will be able to place it on a tray in the oven and keep it warm until they are all done.

4. Eat the warm pancakes immediately with maple syrup and the fruit of your choice - if desired.

5. Banana and Berry Smoothie

Ingredients

- 4 frozen strawberries
- 1 frozen banana
- ½ cup fresh blueberries
- ¼ cup apple juice
- 1 scoop of a Vegan Protein powder

Instructions

Simply mix all the ingredients together in an electric blender until you have a smooth consistency. Pour into a glass and enjoy!

1. It is possible to make this with any fruit or even to add in a few vegetables for added flavor or protein. Experimenting with different mixtures is important.

Pumpkin Bread

Ingredients

- ½ cup water
- ½ cup canned pumpkin
- 5 tbsp. orange juice
- 1 tbsp canola oil
- 1 tbsp maple syrup
- 1 ½ cups whole wheat flour
- 1 cup bread flour
- 1 tbsp powdered soy milk
- Pinch salt
- 1 tsp pumpkin pie spice
- Small amount of orange zest
- active dry yeast
- ¼ cup golden raisins – if required

Instructions

1. Firstly whisk together the water and the pumpkin place this mixture into the bread pan and add the orange juice, oil, and syrup.

Next, add the whole wheat flour, bread flour, soy milk, salt, pumpkin pie spice and orange zest to the bread pan. These ingredients will sit on the top of the wet mixture and you will be able to make a dip in the surface with either your finger of the back of a spoon. Place the yeast in this dip.

2. The bread can then be cooked in bread machine; set the program for a small loaf and leave it to mix. If you would like to add raisins this should be done after the mixing has been completed and before the kneading cycle starts. Once the machine has finished you will have some delicious, vegan bread.

3. Whilst still warm cover with your choice of topping and enjoy.

7. Tofu 'Eggs'

Ingredients

- 1 block tofu - drained and pressed; ideally this should be the extra firm tofu. Remember the firmer the tofu the higher the protein count.
- 1 tbsp yellow mustard
- ¼ tbsp turmeric

Instructions

1. Take two or three large scoops of tofu, preferably with a large melon baller, if you do not have a melon baller then a large tablespoon should be used. The tofu should be pressed into semicircles; this will ensure they look like an egg cut in half.

2. Next, with either a small melon baller or a teaspoon, gently create a small pocket in the flat side of your "eggs"

3. The tofu which has been removed from the "eggs" should be mixed with the turmeric and the mustard. If you need

more tofu take some from the original block.

Mix the ingredients and slowly mash them; add more turmeric and mustard if required to create the color and consistency of a hardboiled egg yolk. Again, this can also be adapted to your own taste preference.
4. Place the turmeric mixture into the pockets of the "eggs" and serve with some whole wheat toast.

8. Chorizo" Breakfast Tacos

Ingredients:
- 8 6-inch corn tortillas
- 2 tbsp olive oil
- 1 red onion - chopped
- 1 tbsp chopped garlic
- Pinch of salt

- Fresh ground black pepper
- 1 ½ blocks of firm tofu
- 1 red pepper - chopped
- 1 tbsp chili powder
- 2 limes - 1 halved and 1 quartered
- ¼ cup chopped fresh cilantro to garnish
- ¼ cup chopped scallions to garnish

Directions:

1. Place all the tortillas onto a large square of foil and loosely wrap them.

2. Preheat the oven to 400.

3. Put a little oil in a skillet and warm, then, add the onion and garlic. You can also season with a little salt and pepper, according to your tastes.

4. Keep on a medium heat and cook the mixture whilst stirring. The vegetables should soften within a few minutes.

5. Crumble the tofu into the pan, ideally this should be done by hand but if this is not possible gently break it apart in separate bowl with a fork.

6. Keep the mixture on the heat and stir continuously, making sure none of the mixture sticks to the pan. The tofu will brown within approximately ten minutes although you can cook it for longer depending upon your personal tastes. The longer you cook it the crisper it will become. When you have nearly finished preparing the tofu put your pre-wrapped tortillas in the oven.

7. Finally add the pepper to your pan and sprinkle some chili powder into the mix. Stir and continue to cook for a further minute.

8. Spread the mix onto your warm tortillas and squeeze the juice from one of the limes all over them.

9. If required, garnish with cilantro and scallions and the lime quarters.

9. Banana and Blueberry Bars

Ingredients

- 1 cup of dates, pitted and halved
- 1½ cups apple juice
- 3 cups rolled oats
- ¾ tsp ground cinnamon
- ¼ tsp ground nutmeg
- 1 ½ tbsp baking powder
- 1 large banana
- 1 tsp vanilla extract
- 1 cup fresh blueberries
- ½ cup walnuts

Instructions

1. Soak the dates in the apple juice for roughly ten to fifteen minutes.

2. Preheat the oven to 375ºF. Then line a baking pan with parchment paper – it is essential to cover the sides.

3. Mix 2 cups of the rolled oats with the cinnamon, nutmeg, and baking powder. Leave this to one side for a moment.

4. Take the rest of the oats, the bananas, and the vanilla extract and blend. You should now be able to remove the dates from the apple juice and place to one side. Use the juice in your mixture; strain it and add it to the blender. Blend the entire mixture until it is creamy.

5. Next add the dates to the blender, and pulse to ensure the dates are in small pieces.

6. Now mix the banana mixture with the oats, cinnamon and nutmeg. Mix everything together thoroughly and then add in the blueberries and walnuts.

7. Pour the mixture into the pre-prepared baking pan and bake for approximately thirty to thirty five minutes.

8. The bars should be allowed to cool at room temperature for roughly ten minutes before cutting. Serve immediately.

10. Breakfast Burrito

Ingredients

- 3 large potatoes – shredded; they can be peeled or unpeeled according to your preference
- 2 tbsp nutritional yeast
- ½ yellow onion - diced
- 1 red pepper - diced
- 1 zucchini - diced
- 8 white or crimini mushrooms - sliced
- ½ to 1 bunch greens (this can be whatever you have to hand; kale, chard, collards, spinach, etc.)

- Juice from 1 lime
- 2 tsp dried basil
- 1 ½ tsp garlic powder
- 1 ½ tsp oregano
- 1 tsp chili powder
- ½ tsp red pepper flakes
- 1 can diced tomatoes
- 1 can black beans
- 1 can pinto beans
- ½ cup chopped fresh cilantro leaves

Instructions:

1. Place the shredded potatoes in a pan with a steamer basket and one inch of water and cook until soft; this should only take between five and ten minutes. Once cooked separate the potatoes equally into two bowls.

2. In one of the bowls, mix in two tablespoons of nutritional yeast and leave the mixture to one side.

3. Now sauté the onion, pepper, zucchini and mushrooms in two tablespoons of water for 5 minutes, you may need to add additional water to ensure the mixture does not stick.

4. Place all the greens in the pan and cook for a few more minutes until they are soft.

5. Next, mix in the lime juice, dried herbs and spices, 1 tablespoon of nutritional yeast, and the steamed potatoes from earlier which did not have the nutritional yeast added.

6. Remove the mixture from the heat and fold in the tomatoes, beans and cilantro.

7. Spread the mixture evenly into a glass baking dish and evenly apply the

remaining potato-nutritional yeast mixture across the top.

8. Bake at 375º F for thirty five to forty minutes, the topping should be lightly browned around the edges.

9. Let it cool for five minutes before serving. If desired garnish with a few pumpkin seeds.

11. Oat Cookies

Ingredients

- 1 cup rolled oats
- 1 cup oat flour
- ½ cup raisins
- ¼ cup unsweetened finely shredded coconut
- 1 tsp baking powder
- 1 tsp cinnamon
- 1 tsp lemon or orange zest – this can be left out if not desired.
- Pinch of sea salt
- Nutmeg – again this can be left out if not to your taste.
- ½ cup unsweetened applesauce
- ¼ cup pure maple syrup
- 2-3 tbsp non-dairy chocolate chips – if desired

Instructions

1. Preheat the oven to 350°F.
2. Then prepare your baking sheet by lining it with parchment paper.

3. Mix the oats, oat flour, raisins, coconut, baking powder, cinnamon, zest, salt and nutmeg together; you should be sure to stir extremely well.
4. Add the applesauce, maple syrup, and chocolate chips (if required).
5. Continue stirring until all ingredients are blended smoothly together.
6. Place mounds of the mixture onto the baking sheet. Each mound should be roughly the size of a tablespoon
7. Place the baking sheet in the oven and bake for roughly fifteen minutes. Allow the pan to cool for approximately one minute before transferring the cookies to a cooling rack.
8. These are great for breakfast or can be had at anytime of the day as a nutritional treat.

12. Vegan Cheese Omelet

INGREDIENTS

- 200g firm tofu
- ¼ tsp turmeric
- ¼ tsp ground garlic granules
- salt
- 3 tbsp nutritional yeast
- ¾ cup soya milk
- 1 large tsp tahini
- 1 ½ tbsp white flour
- 1 tbsp of chickpea
- 4 slices of your preferred vegan cheese
- Sunflower oil for frying

METHOD

Use an electric hand blender and mix all the ingredients together until you have a smooth consistency

1. Next heat up a little oil in a pan. When it is hot put in one ladle of the mixture and allow it to settle for a few seconds. Make sure that it is evenly distributed.

2. As soon as you have spread the mixture evenly add some of the cheese.

3. Once the cheese has melted fold one half of the omelet on top of itself.

4. Turn the omelet over and allow it to cook for a further minute or two – it should now be a golden color.

5. Serve immediately, have it by itself or with anything else you fancy!

13. **Pumpkin Oatmeal Recipe**

Ingredients

- ½ cup oats
- 1 cup water
- 3 tbsp pumpkin puree
- dash of nutmeg
- ½ tsp cinnamon

- ¼ cup raisins – if desired
- ¼ cup full fat coconut milk

Cooking Directions

Place all the ingredients except for the coconut milk into a pan and mix thoroughly whilst bringing to the boil.
1. Allow the mixture to simmer for five minutes.

2. Pour the mixture into your serving bowl and add the coconut milk.

3. Consume immediately, if desired the raisins can be replaced with blueberries or any other fruit you desire.

14. Basic Scrambled Tofu

This is a basic recipe which you can add all sorts of different flavors too, experiment and find the one you like the most!

Ingredients

- Spice blend:
- 2 tsp ground cumin
- 1 tsp dried thyme
- ½ tsp ground turmeric
- Pinch of salt
- 3 tbsp water
- 2 tbsp olive oil
- 3 cloves garlic - minced (this can be adjusted to your own tastes)
- 1 pound extra-firm tofu – make sure you drain this.
- ¼ cup nutritional yeast
- Fresh black pepper to taste

Instructions

1. Mix the spice blend with the water in a small bowl or cup and put to one side.

2. Preheat a large, heavy bottomed pan and sauté the garlic in olive oil for approximately one minute.

3. Break the tofu into bite sized pieces, as small or large as you wish and sauté for roughly ten minutes - stir often so that it does not stick. All the water should evaporate.

4. Mix in the pre-prepared spice blend and then add the nutritional yeast and fresh black pepper. Cook for a further five minutes and serve immediately.

Feel free to add any mixture you wish to create your own, unique flavor.

15. Vegan Granola Bars

Ingredients

- 1 ½ cups rolled oats
- ½ cup brown sugar
- ½ cup oat flour

- Pinch of salt
- Pinch of cinnamon
- ½ cup dried fruit chopped - mixed or single flavor.
- ½ cup nuts chopped – any variety
- ¼ tahini
- 1 tsp vanilla
- 3 tbsp olive oil
- 1 tbsp water
- natural wax paper

Instructions

- Preheat your oven to 350 and line a pan with the wax paper.

  Start by mixing together all the dry ingredients.
  In a separate bowl mix together all the wet ingredients.

Now thoroughly mix the two bowls together so that all the ingredients are combined

- Pour the mixture into your pan and press it down into all the corners.

- Cook in the preheated oven until it browns slightly at the edges. This should be approximately thirty five to forty minutes.

- Leave the cooked bars in the pan until they are completely cooled. It is then best to chill them for a further hour in the fridge before removing it from the pan and cutting to your required size. Store in a cool, dry place and consume as needed – ideal for breakfast on the go or a mid morning snack!

Chapter 3 – 16 Delicious Lunch Recipes

It is important to eat a filling lunch with a balance of carbohydrates and protein; this will ensure you do not succumb to cravings during the afternoon and that you consume all the necessary nutrients. All the following recipes can be used as lunch or dinner depending upon the time available and where you are at lunch or dinner time.

1. Zucchini noodles with Lemon Avocado Pesto

Zucchini is an excellent alternative to pasta; this recipe tops them with creamy avocado and a pine nut pesto; which takes just five minutes to blend. The meal is delicious, high in protein and low in carbs.

Ingredients:

- 2 zucchini - shredded

- ½ avocado - peeled

- 1 tbsp pine nuts

- ½ clove garlic

- ¼ lemon – it will need to be juiced

- Pinch sea salt

Directions:

1. Use a grater on a food processor and shred the zucchini.

2. Combine all the other ingredients in the food processor until well-blended, it may be necessary to scrape the sides – this is the pesto topping.

3. Mix the pesto into the zucchini noodles. If required you can top with additional pine nuts or more pine nuts.

2. Parsnip Pear Soup

Ingredients:
- 1 tbsp olive oil
- ½ cup diced shallots
- 1 garlic clove
- 1 ½ pounds parsnips - peeled and diced
- 3 pears - diced
- 6 cups low sodium no-chicken broth
- A little thyme
- 2 tbsp maple syrup
- 1 tbsp white wine vinegar
- ¼ tsp salt
- Ground black pepper

Directions:

1. Heat the oil in a soup pot; then add the shallots and garlic. Sauté for one to two minutes until translucent.
2. Stir in the parsnips and cook for approximately two minutes; you can then lower the heat to medium and cover.
3. Cook for a further five minutes - the parsnips should be tender and starting to brown.
4. Stir in the pears and cook for another five minutes, keeping the pan covered.

5. Next add the broth and a little thyme. Bring the mixture to the boil and simmer uncovered for another thirty minutes.

6. Turn off the heat and blend until smooth. Stir in the maple syrup, white wine vinegar, salt and pepper according to your tastes.

3. Crab Cakes

Ingredients:
- ½ cup vegan mayonnaise

- 1 tbsp fresh lemon juice
- 1 tbsp chopped fresh dill
- 1 tsp minced garlic
- grape seed or sunflower oil
- 1 can hearts of palm – this will need to be roughly chopped
- ¼ cup chopped celery
- ¼ cup diced red pepper
- ½ cup chopped onion
- 2 tsp minced garlic
- 2 ½ tbsp Old Bay Seasoning
- 1 tsp cornstarch
- ½ cup gluten-free bread crumbs
- Lemon wedges to garnish – if required

Directions:

Crab Cakes

- Heat oil in a large skillet
- Add the hearts of palm and sauté for 8 to 10 minutes, stirring occasionally to prevent sticking. They should go golden brown on all sides. Leave to cool and then mix the celery and peppers in.
- Heat a little oil in a skillet and add the onions - sauté until translucent, this should take two or three minutes. Add the garlic and sauté for a further minute.
- Remove from the heat and mix the contents of the two skillets together. Add seasoning, cornstarch, and mayo.
- Transfer the mixture to a mixing bowl and ensure it has all been mixed well. This mixture must be left to cool, once it is at room temperature you can shape the mixture into four round patties.

Breading

1. Combine the bread crumbs and seasoning in a bowl. Then coat the

patties with this breadcrumb mixture and refrigerate for twenty minutes.
2. Heat a little oil in a medium sized skillet until the oil is hot. Place the patties carefully in the skillet and cook until golden brown on each side. This should take approximately two minutes for each side. Ideally these should be served hot with the lemon wedges on the side.

4. Mushroom, Corn, and Black Bean Farro

Ingredients:

- 1 cup farro
- 2 cups vegetable broth
- 1 tbsp olive oil
- 1 onion - diced
- 3 cloves garlic – these will need to be minced
- 8oz baby bella mushrooms - sliced
- 2 cups frozen corn

- salt
- freshly ground pepper
- 1 can black beans, drained and rinsed
- ½ cup finely chopped fresh cilantro
- juice of ½ lime

Directions:

1. Combine the farro and broth in a medium saucepan and bring to the boil. Reduce the heat and simmer until all the broth is absorbed.
2. Heat the olive oil in a skillet. Mix the onion and garlic in the skillet and cook until tender; this should take no more than three minutes. Add the mushrooms, cumin and corn, then the salt and pepper according to taste. Cook for a further seven minutes until the mushrooms are soft. Remove the pan from the heat.
3. Next combine the cooked farro, mushroom mixture, black beans, cilantro, and lime juice and toss. This

can be served warm or it can be chilled for an hour and served cold.

5. Kale Quinoa Salad with Red Grapes

Ingredients:
- ¾ tsp sea salt
- 1 cup quinoa
- fresh-squeezed lemon juice
- ½ tsp cumin
- ¼ tsp coriander
- 1 pinch red pepper flakes
- ½ cup extra virgin olive oil
- 2 cups stemmed finely chopped kale
- ¼ cup chopped fresh mint
- ¼ cup chopped parsley
- 1 tsp lemon zest
- ¼ cup halved red seedless grapes

Directions:

1. Rinse the quinoa in a fine-mesh strainer under cold running water.
2. Using a small saucepan, bring a little water and ½ teaspoon of the salt to the boil. Add the quinoa and simmer for fifteen to twenty minutes. Keep the pan covered except for when stirring once halfway through. The quinoa should be just tender. Take the pan of the heat and allow the quinoa to stand for ten minutes. The quinoa will then need fluffing; this can be done with a fork.
3. While the quinoa has been cooking, you will be able to whisk together the lemon juice, a ¼ teaspoon of salt, cumin, coriander, red pepper flakes, and olive oil together. When thoroughly mixed add the kale and wait for the quinoa to be cooled. Next add the cooked quinoa, mint, parsley, lemon zest, and grapes. The whole mixture should be tossed. Serve immediately at room temperature. If you need to store them then ensure you use an airtight container and keep

them in the refrigerator for up to 5 days.

6. White bean salad with olives and arugula

Ingredients:
- 3 tbsp extra-virgin olive oil
- 3 tbsp sesame oil
- 3 tbsp fresh lemon juice
- 3 tbsp sherry wine vinegar
- sea salt
- 2 cans cannellini beans - drained and rinsed
- 2 carrots - sliced
- 1 red pepper - diced
- ½ small chopped red onion
- ¾ cup pitted Kalamata olives - diced
- chopped fresh basil

- 3 cups wild arugula leaves
- 1 cup cherry tomatoes - halved
- ¼ cup toasted sesame seeds
- fresh ground black pepper

Directions:

1. The dressing should be made first in a large bowl, whisk together the olive and sesame oils, lemon juice, vinegar, and salt. Then add the beans, carrots, pepper, onion, olives, and basil. Toss thoroughly to ensure all the ingredients are coated. This mixture can be refrigerated until needed.
3. Just before you serve you will need to add the arugula, tomatoes, and sesame seeds. Salt and pepper may be added according to your tastes

7. Veggie and Hummus Sandwich

Ingredients

- 2 slices whole-grain bread
- 2 tbsp hummus

- 3 slices of cucumber
- 2 slices of tomato
- 3 slices of avocado
- ¼ cup alfalfa sprouts
- ¼ cup grated carrots

Directions

1. Firstly toast the bread.
2. Then, spread one tablespoon of hummus on each slice of bread, add the vegetables in layers and either keep as two open sandwiches or close the two slices together to make a sandwich.

8. Soy-Lime Tofu & Rice Bento Lunch

Ingredients

Tofu & Dipping Sauce

- 1 14-ounce package extra-firm, water-packed tofu, drained
- ¼ cup reduced-sodium soy sauce
- ¼ cup lime juice

- 3 tbsp toasted sesame oil
- 1 tbsp prepared peanut sauce
- 1 tbsp coconut milk

To prepare tofu:

Pat tofu dry and cut into half inch cubes. Combine the soy sauce, lime juice and oil in a shallow dish and add the tofu. Combine the ingredients by gently tossing. Leave the mix to marinate in the refrigerator for between one and four hours; it may need to be gently stirred once or twice.

1. Preheat oven to 450°F.
2. Extract the tofu from its marinating sauce and discard the sauce. Then spread the tofu out on a baking sheet and make sure the pieces do not touch. Roast the tofu until golden brown; this should take about twenty minutes and you should turn them once, halfway through.
3. Finally combine the peanut sauce and coconut milk to make a dipping sauce.

Rice Balls

- ½ cup cooked short-grain brown rice
- 2 tsp rice vinegar
- Pinch of salt
- 2 tbsp black sesame seeds – if required

To prepare rice balls:

1. Mix the rice, vinegar and salt in a bowl and mash using a fork. The mixture should become a little sticky.
2. Damp your hands, then press and squeeze the rice into 4 balls.
3. If required sprinkle each ball with sesame seeds.

Fruit & Vegetables

- 1 cup steamed sugar snap peas
- 6 strawberries, hulled
- 6 orange wedges

These are optional and can be adjusted to your personal preferences, simply serve with the rice balls and tofu.

9. Peanut Tofu Wrap

This is an exceptional quick and surprisingly healthy snack. It can be made with Thai peanut sauce which can be purchased at almost any store. For added flavor simply add a few of your favorite vegetables, this will increase the nutritional value of your lunch.

Ingredients

- 1 tbsp store-bought Thai peanut sauce
- 8-inch whole-wheat flour tortilla
- 2oz sliced seasoned baked tofu
- ¼ cup sliced red pepper
- 8 sliced snow peas

Preparation

1. Spread the peanut sauce on to the tortilla. Then place the tofu, peppers and snow peas in the center. Finish by folding the sides over the filling and rolling the tortilla up

2. If you are likely to be consuming this out it can be helpful to wrap your tortilla up; this will prevent the filling from spilling out whilst you are eating it.

10. Quinoa Salad with Creamy Avocado Dressing

Ingredients

- 1 cup uncooked quinoa
- 1 can black beans, drained and rinsed
- 200grams grape tomatoes
- 1 orange pepper - diced
- 1 large avocado - diced
- ½ cup diced cucumber
- ½ cup sweet corn
- ¼ cup diced red onion
- Salt and pepper if required
- ¼ cup chopped cilantro

Creamy Avocado Dressing

- 1 ripe avocado, peeled and seeded
- ¼ cup silken tofu
- 1 clove garlic - minced
- water

- 2 tbsp chopped cilantro
- 1 tbsp tahini
- 1 tbsp chopped green onion
- 1 tbsp fresh lime juice
- ¼ tsp ground cumin
- ⅛ tsp chili powder
- Salt and ground black pepper, to taste

Instructions

1. Add the quinoa and 2 cups of salted water to a saucepan. Cover and then bring to the boil before reducing the heat to its lowest setting. Allow it to simmer until the water is completely absorbed. The quinoa should be fluffy within twenty minutes.

While the quinoa is cooking you can make the Creamy Avocado Dressing. Mix all the dressing ingredients in a food processor and blend until smooth.

3. Once the quinoa has cooked combine it with the black beans, tomatoes, peppers, avocado, cucumber, corn, red onion. Pour the dressing over the quinoa mixture and stir well until everything is thoroughly coated.

Season with salt and pepper if required. You can also squeeze fresh lime juice over the salad; this will prevent the avocado from going brown. Garnish the salad with chopped cilantro. It can be served at room temperature or chilled for an hour before serving.

11. Coconut Curry Lentil Soup

Ingredients

- 1 tbsp coconut oil (or olive oil)
- 1 large onion, chopped
- 2 cloves garlic, minced
- 1 tbsp fresh ginger, minced
- 2 tbsp tomato paste (or ketchup)
- 2 tbsp curry powder
- ½ tsp hot red pepper flakes
- 4 cups vegetable broth
- 1 400ml can coconut milk
- 1 400g can diced tomatoes
- 1 ½ cups dry red lentils
- 2-3 handfuls of chopped kale or spinach
- salt and pepper - to taste

- Garnish: chopped cilantro and/or vegan sour cream

Instructions

1. Ideally this should be created in a stockpot. The coconut oil should be heated and then the onion, garlic and ginger can be stir fried until the onion is translucent. This should take between two and three minutes.
2. Add the tomato paste (or ketchup), curry powder, and red pepper flakes and cook for a further minute.
3. Then add the vegetable broth, coconut milk, diced tomatoes and lentils. Bring the mixture to the boil, covering the pan whilst doing so. Keep it covered whilst you simmer on a low heat for between twenty and thirty minutes. The lentils should become very tender. If desired you can season with salt and pepper.
4. To add the finishing touches before serving, stir in the kale/spinach and garnish with cilantro and/or vegan sour cream.

12. Easy Lemon Lentil Soup

Ingredients

- 1 tbsp olive oil
- 1 onion, chopped
- 2 cloves garlic, finely chopped
- pinch hot red pepper flakes
- 1 tsp cumin
- 1 ½ cups dry red lentils
- 6 cups vegetable broth
- salt and pepper if required
- 2 tbsp lemon juice
- 2 cups kale or spinach, chopped – if required
- 2 tbsp fresh parsley - finely chopped

Instructions

Heat the oil before adding the onion, pepper flakes and garlic. Cook all the ingredients for five minutes.

1. Add cumin, lentils, broth, salt & pepper and bring the mixture to the boil.
2. Cover the pan and simmer on a low heat until the lentils are tender and the soup is beginning to thicken. This

should be approximately thirty minutes.
3. Stir in lemon juice and kale/spinach if required. You can also add parsley or cilantro.

13. Refreshing Quinoa Salad with Mango, Cucumber, Avocado & Black Beans

Ingredients

- 1 cup quinoa, rinsed and drained
- 1 can black beans, rinsed drained
- 1 fresh mango, cubed
- 1 ripe avocado, cubed
- 1 cucumber - diced
- ½ cup mint, chopped
- ½ cup fresh coriander - chopped
- ⅓ cup olive oil
- 2 tbsp lime juice
- 1 clove garlic
- salt and pepper if required

Instructions

1. Two cups of salted water need to be added to the quinoa and brought to the boil in a saucepan. The pan should be covered and left to simmer for approximately twenty minutes until all the water is absorbed and the quinoa is fluffy.
2. Next, whisk together the olive oil, lime juice, and garlic.

Finally add all the ingredients together; including the quinoa, and gently combine. Season with salt and pepper if required. It is best served chilled, after twenty minutes in the fridge.

14. Grilled Mediterranean Vegetables on White Bean Mash

Ingredients

- 1 red pepper - quartered
- 1 aubergine - sliced lengthways
- 2 courgettes - sliced lengthways
- 2 tbsp olive oil

For the Mash

- 410g can haricot beans - rinsed
- 1 garlic clove , crushed
- 100ml vegetable stock
- 1 tbsp chopped coriander
- lemon wedges, to garnish if required

Instructions

1. Place all the vegetables in a grill pan and brush them lightly with oil. Grill on a medium heat until they turn light brown, then turn them over and brush the other side with a little oil. Grill again until tender.
2. The beans should be placed into a small pan with the garlic and the stock. Bring the pan to the boil before simmering uncovered for approximately ten minutes. Mash the beans roughly with a potato masher; if necessary add a little water or more stock if the mixture is too dry.
3. The mash and vegetables should be placed onto two plates and any leftover oil can be drizzled on top. If required add a sprinkle of black pepper and

coriander. Add a lemon wedge to each plate and serve.

15. Cauliflower and Lentil Coconut Curry

Ingredients

- 2 tbsp vegetable oil
- 1 onion, finely chopped
- 1 garlic clove, minced
- 2.5 cm piece fresh ginger, peeled and grated
- 2 tsp ground coriander
- 2 tsp ground cumin
- ½ tsp ground turmeric
- ⅓ cup dry red lentils
- 250 ml vegetable broth, hot
- 1 head cauliflower, cut into small florets
- 1 large carrot - diced
- 400 ml can coconut milk
- ¾ cup frozen green beans or peas, thawed and drained

- 2 tbsp chopped fresh
- 1 tbsp lemon juice
- salt and freshly ground black pepper to taste

Instructions

1. Heat 1½ tbsp of oil and gently cook the onion for ten minutes on a medium heat. They should be stirred frequently until they are soft and translucent. Then add the garlic, ginger, coriander, cumin and turmeric and cook for a further two minutes.
2. Add the lentils to the mixture and pour in the broth. Bring the mixture to the boil, before reducing the heat. Keep the pan covered and leave it to simmer for approximately ten minutes.
3. Whilst the lentils are simmering heat the remaining oil in a frying pan and fry the cauliflower for two or three minutes until lightly browned. Then add the cauliflower, carrot and coconut milk to the lentil mixture.

4. Bring the mixture back to a gentle simmer and cook for a further ten minutes, or until the vegetables are tender. Add the beans and peas and cook for three to four minutes.
5. Finally stir in 2 tbsp of cilantro and the lemon juice. Flavor the mixture with a little salt and freshly ground black pepper as required. Garnish with a little additional cilantro.

16. Healthy Vegan Quinoa Chili

Ingredients

- 2 cups vegetable stock
- 1 cup quinoa - rinsed well
- 1 tbsp olive oil
- 1 large onion - diced
- 2 cloves garlic - minced
- 2 celery stalks - diced
- 1 carrot - diced
- 1 red pepper - diced
- 400g diced tomatoes with juices

- 420g kidney beans, NOT drained
- 1 tsp chili powder
- ½ tsp dried oregano
- ½ tsp ground cumin
- salt & freshly ground pepper to taste
- 1 cup corn kernels (drained if using canned)

Instructions

1. Put the vegetable stock in a saucepan and bring to the boil. Then add the quinoa, cover the pan and simmer on your lowest setting until ready. This should take about fifteen minutes. It is ready when curls start to appear out of the grains.
2. Heat the olive oil in a large saucepan. Then add the onions and garlic, and sauté until tender; this should take approximately three minutes. Finally add the celery and carrot – this mixture should be cooked until tender; approximately another three minutes.
3. Add the pepper, tomatoes, kidney beans, chili powder, oregano and

cumin. If required put a little salt and pepper in the pan. Bring everything to the boil and then simmer for approximately thirty minutes, stirring occasionally. The pan should be kept uncovered. After thirty minutes stir in the quinoa and corn.
4. This dish is best served topped with diced avocado, tofu sour cream, cilantro and a little shredded cucumber. To finish add a side of corn chips or cornbread.

Chapter 4 – 10 Delightful Dinner Recipes

1. Curried Coconut Quinoa with Roasted Cauliflower

Ingredients

- 1 head cauliflower, cut into bite-sized florets
- 3 tbsp melted coconut oil
- cayenne pepper to taste
- Sea salt to taste
- 1 onion - chopped
- 1 tsp ground ginger
- 1 tsp ground turmeric
- ½ tsp curry powder of choice
- ½ teaspoon ground cardamom
- 1 can light coconut milk
- ½ cup water
- 1 cup quinoa - rinsed well

- ⅓ cup raisins

- 1 tbsp apple cider vinegar

- 4 cups baby arugula or spinach

Instructions

1. Preheat your oven to 425 degrees Fahrenheit.

2. Lightly toss the cauliflower florets with the coconut oil, cayenne pepper and a light sprinkle of sea salt. Then roast for thirty minutes in the middle of the oven, you will need to turn them after fifteen minutes. The cauliflower should be tender golden.

3. You will need a pot with a lid; warm some coconut oil until hot and then add the onion and cook for about 5 minutes. Add the ginger, turmeric, curry powder and cardamom and stir until fragrant; this should only take approximately thirty seconds.

4. Pour in the coconut milk, water, rinsed quinoa and raisins. Then slowly bring the

mixture to the boil and allow it to simmer for fifteen minutes.

5. Allow the mixture to cool for five minutes before fluffing the quinoa with a fork.

6. Stir in the salt, vinegar, arugula and spinach.

7. Serve immediately with the roasted cauliflower on top.

2. Sweet Potato & Black Bean Veggie Burgers

Ingredients

- 1½ pounds sweet potatoes
- ⅓ cup uncooked millet or quinoa
- 1 cup oats
- 1 can black beans, rinsed and drained
- ½ red onion - diced

- ½ cup lightly packed fresh cilantro leaves, chopped
- 2 tsp cumin powder
- 1 tsp chili powder
- 1 tsp chipotle powder
- cayenne powder
- salt
- Sunflower oil or coconut oil
- 8 whole wheat hamburger buns

Instructions

1. Preheat the oven to 400 degrees Fahrenheit.

2. Slice the sweet potatoes lengthwise and place them cut side down on a baking sheet. Bake them until you can gently squeeze them – this should be approximately thirty to forty minutes but this will depend upon the size of the potato.

3. Wait until the potatoes are cool enough to handle and then pull the skin off before roughly chopping the inside. They can then be left to cool.

4. Bring one cup of water to the boil in a saucepan and then stir in the millet. Allow this to simmer for approximately twenty five minutes; until it is tender.

5. Drain off any liquid which has not been absorbed or evaporated and leave to cool.

6. The oats need to be ground; it is easiest to use a food processor or blender. Make sure they are broken up without becoming as fine as flour.

   Using your electric mixer combine the cooled sweet potatoes and millet with the black beans, onion, cilantro, cumin, chili powder, chipotle or paprika, cayenne and salt. Mix all the ingredients thoroughly; it should have the consistency of mash.

7. Next add the ground oats into the mixture and stir well. You should be able to form a patty which stays together.

8. If time allows chill the mixture for an hour – the patties will stay together better.

9. Gently shape half a cup of the mixture into a patty about 3½ inches in diameter. Gently flatten to create a smooth burger; the mixture should create eight burgers.

10. To cook the burgers heat 1 tablespoon of oil in a skillet and place several of the burgers into the pan. You will need to cook each side for approximately three or four minutes until they are brown.

11. If you wish to toast the buns put them on a baking sheet, cut sides up, and bake for two or three minutes.

3. Chopped Kale Salad with Edamame, Carrot and Avocado

Ingredients

- 1 bunch kale

- sea salt

- 1 cup chopped snow peas

- 1 large carrot
- 1 small red pepper - chopped
- 1 heaped cup organic edamame
- 1 avocado, pitted and sliced into small chunks
- 1 large shallot - sliced
- cilantro
- basil - chopped

Tamari-Ginger Vinaigrette
- ¼ cup olive oil
- 2 tbsp rice vinegar
- 1 tbsp finely grated ginger
- 1 tbsp low-sodium tamari
- 2 tsp lime juice
- 3 garlic cloves - minced

Instructions
1. Remove the tough ribs from the kale and discard them.

2. Chop the kale leaves into bite-sized pieces before placing them into a mixing bowl.

3. Sprinkle the kale with a little sea salt, according to taste and scrunch the leaves with your hands until the kale is dark green and fragrant.

   Add all the other salad ingredients and mix thoroughly.

   For the vinaigrette, whisk together all the ingredients until emulsified.

4. Then simply serve the salad with the dressing drizzled all over it.

4. Spicy Roasted Ratatouille with Spaghetti

Ingredients

- 2 pints cherry or grape tomatoes
- 1 eggplant - diced
- 1 zucchini - diced
- 1 yellow squash - diced
- 1 red pepper - diced

- 1 onion - diced
- 6 tbsp olive oil
- 2 tbsp balsamic vinegar
- 6 cloves garlic – minced
- salt
- Freshly ground black pepper
- Red pepper flakes
- ½ pound whole grain spaghetti
- 2 tbsp chopped fresh basil
- 1 tbsp chopped fresh oregano
- 1 tsp fresh thyme

Instructions
1. Preheat the oven to 425 degrees Fahrenheit and ensure you able to access both the middle positions.

2. Using a small baking dish cover the whole baby tomatoes with 2 tablespoons olive oil and a sprinkle of salt and pepper.

3. In a separate bowl thoroughly mix the diced eggplant, zucchini, yellow squash, bell pepper and onion.

4. Then whisk together ¼ cup olive oil, the balsamic vinegar, garlic, salt, and a few generous twists of black pepper and a pinch of red pepper flakes. (according to your preference)

5. Drizzle it over the vegetables ensuring they are all covered completely.

6. Arrange the vegetables in a single layer on a baking sheet and put in the middle part of the oven for twenty minutes. At the same time place the tomatoes in the lower part of the oven

7. Whilst this is cooking bring a large pot of salted water to the boil and cook the pasta until al dente. Drain the pasta and save one cup of the cooking water.

8. After 20 minutes the tomatoes will be ready but the vegetables will need to be turned and cooked for a further ten minutes.

9. Add the tomatoes and their juices to the spaghetti in a serving bowl. Add a splash of the pasta cooking water to the serving bowl and stir to ensure all the pasta is coated in a light tomato sauce.

   Once the vegetables are cooked add them to the bowl and toss lightly to mix all the ingredients.
10. To finish sprinkle with the chopped fresh herbs and season with additional salt, pepper and red pepper flakes – according to your tastes.

5. Butternut Squash Chipotle Chili with Avocado

Ingredients

- 1 red onion - chopped
- 2 red peppers - chopped
- 1 small butternut squash - peeled and chopped

- 4 garlic cloves - minced
- 2 tbsp olive oil
- ground sea salt
- 1 tbsp chili powder
- 1 tsp ground cumin
- ½ tbsp chopped chipotle pepper in
- 1 bay leaf
- ¼ tsp ground cinnamon
- 1 can diced tomatoes, including the liquid
- 4 cups cooked black beans
- 1 can vegetable broth
- 2 Avocados - diced
- 3 corn tortillas for crispy tortilla strips
- cilantro

Instructions

1. You will need to use a stockpot Place the chopped vegetables (onion, bell pepper,

butternut squash, garlic) with two tablespoons of olive oil in the stockpot and warm, stirring regularly to ensure everything cooks thoroughly.

Once cooked lower the heat and add all of the spices and canned ingredients. Stir thoroughly before covering for approximately one hour – it should still be stirred occasionally.

2. Next stack the corn tortillas and slice them into thin strips, each one should be roughly 2 inches long. Add a drizzle of olive oil to a warm pan and put in the tortilla slices, sprinkle them with salt as required and cook until crispy. This should take between four and seven minutes

3. To serve dish the chili into individual bowls and sprinkle the crispy tortilla strips on top with plenty of diced avocado.

6. Creamy Roasted Brussels Sprout and Quinoa Gratin

Ingredients

- 2 cups vegetable broth
- 1 cup quinoa
- 1 pound Brussels sprouts
- 2 tbsp extra-virgin olive oil
- 1 tbsp dried oregano
- 1½ tsp dried thyme
- salt
- freshly ground black pepper
- Pinch of ground nutmeg
- Pinch red pepper flakes
- 4 ounces vegan cheese
- 1 cup almond milk
- ½ tbsp extra-virgin olive oil

- 1 tsp minced garlic
- 1 slice whole wheat bread

Instructions

1. Preheat oven to 375 degrees Fahrenheit.

2. Put the vegetable broth into a heavy bottom pan and bring to the boil. Add the quinoa and simmer for approximately twenty minutes. This can be set aside until later.

3. Cut the Brussels sprouts into halves or quarters and coat them with a little olive oil. Place them in a single layer on a baking sheet and put them in the oven for approximately fifteen minutes.

4. Reduce the oven heat to 350 degrees.

5. Thoroughly stir the dried oregano, thyme, salt, pepper, nutmeg and red pepper flakes into the quinoa. Next add the cheese and stir until it's all melted. Add the milk and ensure the mixture is thoroughly combined.

6. Next stir the Brussels sprouts into the quinoa mix and place the entire mixture onto a baking dish.

7. Cover the mixture with the bread, which has been broken into crumbs in a blender and soaked in a little oil and garlic on a hot stove for a few minutes.

8. Cook in the oven for approximately twenty five minutes. Before serving allow the dish to cool for five or ten minutes.

7. Three Bean Chili with Spring Pesto

Ingredients

- 1 tbsp and ¼ cup extra-virgin olive oil
- 1 onion - chopped
- 2 carrots - diced
- 1 can diced tomatoes, including liquid
- salt and black pepper
- 1 can chickpeas - rinsed and drained
- 1 can cannellini beans - rinsed and drained
- 1 can kidney beans - rinsed and drained
- 1 clove garlic - finely chopped
- 3 tbsp pine nuts - chopped

- 1 cup fresh parsley - chopped
- crusty bread – if required

Directions

1. Place one tablespoon of the oil in a pan and heat, once hot add the onion and carrots. Cook for five minutes, until they are tender.

2. Add the tomatoes in their liquid, 2 cups water, 1 ½ teaspoons salt, and ½ teaspoon pepper. Stir thoroughly and bring the mixture to the boil.

3. Next, add the chickpeas and cannellini and kidney beans and cook thoroughly. The mixture should be heated right the way through; this will take approximately five minutes.

4. Mix the garlic, pine nuts, parsley, and the remaining ¼ cup oil with a little salt and pepper – this will be the pesto topping.

5. Dish the chili into the required number of individual bowls and top with the pesto.

6. Add bread if required.

8. Swiss Chard with Chickpeas and Couscous

Ingredients

- 1 10oz box couscous
- ½ cup pine nuts
- 3 tbsp olive oil
- 2 cloves sliced garlic
- 1 can chickpeas - rinsed
- ½ cup raisins
- 2 bunches Swiss chard – trim the stems
- Salt
- black pepper

Directions

1. Add 1 ½ cups boiling water to a bowl of couscous and stir. Once thoroughly mixed cover and allow them to stand for ten minutes.

2. Using a large pan or skillet heat the pine nuts. It is essential to shake the pan regularly. Within three or four minutes the

nuts will be golden. Put these aside until later.

3. Return the pan or skillet to the heat and add the oil. Once it is hot add the garlic and cook for one minute.

4. Mix in the chickpeas, raisins, chard, salt, and pepper. Continue to heat for approximately five minutes, until the chard is tender.

5. Finally fluff the couscous with a fork and spread it equally onto the individual plates. Garnish by topping with the chard and pine nuts.

9. Linguine with Caper and Green Olive Sauce

Ingredients

- 1 tbsp olive oil
- 2 cloves of sliced garlic
- ¼ tsp crushed red pepper flakes
- 1 jar marinara sauce
- 1 jar Spanish olives- chopped
- 1 jar capers - roughly chopped

- ½ cup fresh parsley
- ½ tsp lemon zest
- 1 box linguine

Directions

1. Place the oil, garlic, and crushed red pepper in a large saucepan and heat for approximately two minutes

2. Mix in the marinara sauce, olives, capers, parsley, and lemon zest and allow it to simmer for fifteen minutes.

3. Whilst this is simmering cook the linguine according to its instructions.

4. Drain and mix the linguine with the sauce before transfer to a serving dish.

5. Serve immediately with some pumpkin bread for additional flavor.

10. Baked Macaroni and Cheese

Ingredients

- 1 lb pasta
- 3 tbsp Vegan butter

- 3 tbsp chickpea flour
- 3 cup soy or almond milk
- Salt and pepper to taste
- ½ tsp paprika
- 1 tbsp spicy brown mustard
- 3 cup cheddar-flavored Daiya
- ½ cup regular or gluten-free bread crumbs
- 2 tsp olive oil
- Canola oil spray

Preparation

1. Preheat your oven to 350 degrees.
2. Fill a large pot with water and a pinch of salt then bring it to the boil and add the pasta. Cook for a few minutes under the time they instructions state. It will finish cooking in the oven.
3. Next melt the Vegan spread in a pan and then add the flour and whisk thoroughly.

Leave on the heat for one minute to allow the flour to cook.

4. Slowly add the milk to the mixture whilst whisking continuously.

5. Next add the salt, pepper, and paprika. The sauce should be left to cook as it will thicken after it has reached boiling point.

6. Drain the pasta and place it back into either the same pan or a new bowl, ready for mixing.

7. You should now add the Daiya to the sauce and stir well until it is melted.

8. Finally add the mustard; you may need to add more milk. The less milk you have the thicker the sauce.

9. Now mix the sauce and the pasta, stirring them together thoroughly.

10. Your macaroni cheese can be served and eaten now or baked as follows:

11. Spray the canola spray onto a baking dish and then fill the dish with the pour the

macaroni and sauce mix; it should naturally form an even layer.

12. Separately mix the bread crumbs and the olive oil to make a fine crumble. Spread this on top of the macaroni and sauce prior to baking. Within thirty minutes the top will be golden brown and bubbling. Now it is ready to serve!

Chapter 5 – 10 Revitalizing Meal Plans

It can often seem that the most delicious looking recipes will require some time to prepare and enjoy. There is a place and a time for this kind of food but it is also essential to be able to produce food quickly whilst staying within the parameters of a vegan lifestyle. The following list shows ten suggestions for a quick breakfast, lunch or dinner; these meals will provide you with all the essential vitamins and minerals you require on a daily basis - including protein. Each of the following can be purchased ready-made, put together quickly at home or pre-prepared and frozen for when you are in a rush.

Breakfast

Oatmeal with walnuts and raisins (most commercial oatmeal is vegan)

Fresh fruit

Soy Yoghurt

Cereal with soy milk

Fresh bagel with non dairy cream cheese

Tofu Scramble

Vegan French toast

Fruit Smoothie

Coconut Latte smoothie

Banana muffins

Lunch

Avocado ReubenSumptuous Spinach Salad with Orange-Sesame Dressing

Carrot & Ginger soup

Tofu Salad

Tofu, lettuce, tomato and avocado salad

Potato and Leek soup

Pasta salad

Italian eggplant sandwich

Apple-pecan pancakes

Vegan cheese salad

Dinner

Tofu-Spinach Lasagna

Fresh tossed salad

Roasted vegetable whole wheat pasta

Vegan Chili – this can be purchased ready-made and is excellent when you have no time to spare.

Vegan Buffalo Wings with baked French fries

Stir fried tofu with vegetables

Risotto with sun dried tomatoes

Humus with pita wedges and your choice of vegetables

Baked Macaroni cheese

Vegan burger and green beans

Conclusion

Adopting a vegan lifestyle is not as difficult as it may at first appear, this book should have provided you with a wide variety of options which will assist you whether you are just starting out in the vegan lifestyle or have been a committed vegan for many years. It is important to understand the importance of vitamins, minerals and the other nutrients which keep your body healthy. Understanding where to obtain these nutrients will enable you to enjoy your food and remain healthy, whilst supporting the environment and protecting all life forms from harm.

Being a vegan is now recognized by the mainstream diet and health professionals and there are health benefits associated with consuming only plant based products. Adopting a vegan lifestyle offers the benefit of knowing that you are at one with nature. This book will also be useful to demonstrate to your friends and relatives that cooking the vegan way does not need to be arduous and they can still prepare a fine meal for you!

The recipes and meal plans suggested in here can all be adjusted and personalized according to your own tastes. As with any cooking it is essential to experiment; it is the only way of finding out what works and what doesn't. Not eating meat can also save you money as meat tends to be one of the more expensive items in the weekly shop. It has to be a satisfying feeling to know you can help the environment and save yourself money in the process!

Whilst no-one wants to force their own beliefs onto other people, you may be surprised by how much others enjoy the variety of food, tastes and flavors which you are able to offer them. This may well make them think twice about the idea of a vegan lifestyle; it is becoming increasingly popular with various celebrities to adopt a vegan lifestyle during the day. Add this to the fact that the vegan diet is now being recognized as low in fat and high in fiber and antioxidants and you can see why so many people are changing the way they eat.

About the Author

Julio Barr is author of several cookbooks on vegan diet. He has written research papers on the topic and currently lives in California.

www.ingramcontent.com/pod-product-compliance
Lightning Source LLC
LaVergne TN
LVHW011944070526
838202LV00054B/4789